BELLY FAT BREAKTHROUGH: SECRETS TO A FLAT STOMACH

The Ultimate Strategies for Losing Abdominal Weight & Reclaiming your health

Dr. Louis Robins

TABLE OF CONTENTS

<u>Foreword by ' Lisa Beattie, Psy.D.'</u>
<u>licensed counseling psychologist</u>

In "Belly Fat Breakthrough: Secrets to a Flat Stomach," renowned health and fitness expert Dr. Louis Robins, delves into the often underestimated and ignored issue of excess belly fat. With an extensive background in nutrition and fitness, Dr. Louis brings a wealth of knowledge to this comprehensive guide that explores the negative impacts of belly fat, its underlying causes, and practical methods for shedding those extra inches around your midsection.

Belly fat, also known as visceral fat, is not just a cosmetic concern; it's a serious health issue. Dr. Louis begins by elucidating the various health risks associated with excess belly fat. From an increased risk of heart disease and type 2 diabetes to hormonal imbalances and reduced mobility, this book uncovers the multifaceted threats that come with that stubborn spare tire.

The book meticulously dissects the causes of belly fat, going beyond the usual suspects of overeating and lack of exercise. Dr. Louis emphasizes the importance of genetics, hormonal imbalances, stress, and even sleep patterns in contributing to abdominal obesity. Readers will gain a deep understanding of why this type of fat can be so challenging to lose and why it's crucial to address the root causes.

But "Belly Fat" doesn't just stop at highlighting the problem. Dr. Louis provides a plethora of practical, evidence-based solutions for tackling belly fat head-on. His comprehensive approach covers a wide range of topics, including nutrition, exercise, stress management, and sleep optimization. He offers readers tailored advice to fit their individual needs, ensuring that everyone can find an approach that suits their lifestyle and goals.

This book features a variety of exercise routines, from targeted abdominal workouts to full-body exercises that help burn fat more effectively. Dr. Louis also presents a range of dietary recommendations, including meal plans, recipes, and guidance on portion control. His emphasis on the importance of a balanced and sustainable approach sets this book apart from fad diet trends, making it a practical and long-term solution.

One of the book's standout features is its focus on the psychological and emotional aspects of weight loss. Dr. Louis addresses the mental challenges and obstacles that often accompany efforts to shed belly fat. He offers strategies for cultivating a positive mindset, setting achievable goals, and maintaining motivation throughout the journey, another important aspect that sets "Belly Fat Breakthrough: Secrets to a Flat Stomach," apart is its exploration of the gut microbiome's role in managing belly fat. Recent research has unveiled the intricate interplay between gut bacteria and obesity. The book elucidates the pivotal connection between the gut microbiome and belly fat, highlighting the link between a balanced gut flora and a slimmer waistline. Readers will discover how certain strains of beneficial bacteria can positively influence metabolism and fat storage, and how to leverage this knowledge for their own benefit.

With his expertise, Dr. Louis guides readers on a transformative journey towards a healthier and happier life. By following the principles outlined in "Belly Fat Breakthrough: Secrets to a Flat Stomach," readers will not only discover the detrimental impacts of belly fat but also acquire the tools and knowledge necessary to effectively reduce it and improve their overall well-being.

In this enlightening and comprehensive guide, Dr. Louis equips readers with the insights and strategies needed to combat belly fat, empowering them to reclaim their health, confidence, and vitality. Whether you're looking to shed a few inches or embark on a life-changing transformation, this book is your trusted companion on the journey to a slimmer, healthier you

INTRODUCTION

Overview of Belly Fat and its Negative Impacts on Humans

The term "belly fat" is a commonly discussed subject, referring to a specific type of fat that accumulates in the abdominal area, often called abdominal or visceral fat. It resides deep within the belly, enveloping crucial organs like the intestines, liver, and pancreas. There are several methods to assess belly fat, but the two most widely used are the waist-to-hip ratio and waist circumference. A prominent indicator of excessive visceral fat is an enlarged waist circumference, especially when it exceeds 40 inches for men and 35 inches for women. Beyond its aesthetic concerns, belly fat carries a multitude of health risks that demand serious consideration.

Before delving further into this topic, I'd like to share a poignant anecdote about my dear friend Anna, whose life was profoundly impacted by abdominal fat. Anna, once a vibrant and cheerful lady, began grappling with an increasing accumulation of belly fat over the years. Initially, it appeared to be primarily a cosmetic issue, but it soon became evident that it was severely affecting her overall health.

Anna's previously lively personality began to wane. Mundane tasks became challenging, and she consistently felt the burden of abdominal heaviness. The additional weight placed pressure on her back, leading to posture problems and discomfort. As her belly expanded, it compressed her diaphragm, making it harder for her to breathe comfortably.

This surplus belly fat triggered a cascade of health issues. She noticed a rise in blood pressure, and a diagnosis of insulin resistance put her at risk for type 2 diabetes. Her joints bore the brunt of the excess weight, resulting in pain and limited mobility. The fat around her belly hindered circulation to her legs, causing constant heaviness and sluggishness.

As the years passed, Anna's health deteriorated further. She was no longer able to engage in the activities she once enjoyed, and she became increasingly isolated. The weight of her abdominal fat weighed on her emotionally and physically, serving as a constant reminder of her diminishing energy and the life she had once led.

This story serves as a poignant reminder of the detrimental effects of excess abdominal fat on individuals. It goes beyond mere appearance; it profoundly impacts general health and well-being. Anna's experience underscores the importance of maintaining a healthy weight, not only for aesthetic reasons but also to preserve one's vitality and quality of life.

To delve into this topic further, it's important to understand that there are two major categories of belly fat:

Subcutaneous fat: This type of fat can be found throughout the body, including the abdomen, and is situated just beneath the skin. Comprising fat cells (adipocytes) and connective tissue, subcutaneous fat serves various essential functions, such as protecting internal organs, storing energy, providing insulation, and contributing to the body's shape and appearance. Subcutaneous fat is relatively flexible and tends to "jiggle" around the abdomen, particularly in women. It's noteworthy that subcutaneous fat is not as strongly linked to an increased risk of diseases as the fat located deeper in the abdominal cavity.

However, it's crucial to recognize that excess body fat, including an accumulation of fat in the abdominal region, can elevate the risk of developing chronic conditions, including:

❖ Weight-related health risks: While a certain amount of subcutaneous fat is necessary and beneficial, an excess, especially when concentrated in the abdomen and upper body, can lead to obesity. Obesity is associated with a range of health issues, including heart disease, high blood pressure, stroke, specific types of cancer, and breathing problems like sleep apnea, where breathing intermittently stops and starts during sleep.

❖ Joint stress: Carrying surplus subcutaneous fat places additional strain on joints, especially in the lower part of the body. This can result in joint discomfort, reduced mobility, and an elevated risk of conditions like osteoarthritis.

❖ Psychological impact: Excessive subcutaneous fat can have adverse effects on an individual's self-esteem and body image, potentially leading to psychological issues such as depression and anxiety.

In summary, while subcutaneous fat serves important bodily functions, an excess of it, particularly in the context of obesity, can lead to significant health drawbacks, including an increased risk of chronic diseases and negative impacts on physical and mental well-being.

Visceral fat: This is the second type of belly fat, it's also known as intra-abdominal or organ fat. It represents a form of fatty tissue stored deep within the abdominal cavity, encompassing and providing cushioning for vital organs such as the liver, pancreas, and intestines. Unlike subcutaneous fat, which resides just beneath the skin, visceral fat is located internally within the body. It is often referred to as "harmful" abdominal fat. In comparison to subcutaneous fat, visceral fat is significantly more metabolically active, containing a higher number of cells, blood vessels, and nerves. While a certain amount of visceral fat is necessary for normal physiological functions, excessive amounts can lead to various health issues, including:

❖ Heightened Health Risks: Excessive visceral fat is closely associated with an increased risk of severe chronic health conditions, including heart disease, type 2 diabetes, and high blood pressure. This fat is metabolically active and releases free fatty acids into the bloodstream, disrupting insulin's ability to regulate blood sugar levels and increasing insulin resistance in various tissues, including muscles and the liver.

* ❖ Inflammatory Effects: Visceral fat releases proinflammatory substances known as cytokines, including tumor necrosis factor-alpha (TNF-alpha) and interleukin-6 (IL-6). Chronic, low-level inflammation is a hallmark of excess visceral fat, and this inflammation is linked to insulin resistance. This inflammation can interfere with insulin's normal signaling pathways and its ability to facilitate glucose uptake into cells. Moreover, visceral fat influences the generation of various bioactive molecules referred to as adipokines. Some adipokines can have adverse effects on insulin sensitivity. For example, adiponectin, a hormone produced by adipose tissue, is typically associated with improved insulin sensitivity, but its levels tend to be lower in individuals with excess visceral fat. Visceral fat is not merely a passive energy storage site; it acts as an active endocrine organ, producing pro-inflammatory substances. As mentioned earlier, it releases various molecules, including pro-inflammatory cytokines like TNF-alpha, IL-6, and C-reactive protein (CRP), initiating and sustaining an inflammatory response. Visceral fat also has the capability to attract immune cells, such as

macrophages, which migrate to the fat tissue. Once within the fat tissue, these macrophages become activated and release more inflammatory cytokines. The infiltration of immune cells is a primary driver of inflammation in visceral fat. The persistent and chronic inflammation associated with visceral fat can extend beyond the fat tissue itself and affect distant organs and tissues, contributing to systemic inflammation, which can be a factor in various health issues, including atherosclerosis, the accumulation of plaque in the arteries.

❖ Disruption of Hormonal Balance: Excess visceral fat can disrupt hormonal balance through a combination of factors, including its metabolic activity and its influence on other hormones and bodily tissues. Some of these factors include:

Release of Adipokines: Fat tissue, including visceral fat, releases a range of bioactive substances known as adipokines. Some of these adipokines play a role in regulating hormones. For instance, excess visceral fat can lead to the overproduction of resistin, which is linked to insulin resistance and inflammation.

Diminished Adiponectin: Adiponectin is a significant adipokine with anti-inflammatory and insulin-enhancing properties. In individuals with an excess of visceral fat, adiponectin levels tend to decrease, potentially resulting in insulin resistance and disruptions in metabolism.

Elevated Leptin Levels: Leptin, a hormone produced by fat cells, plays a role in appetite and metabolism. Excess visceral fat can lead to heightened levels of leptin, potentially causing leptin resistance. When the body becomes resistant to leptin, it can interfere with appetite control, potentially leading to overeating and weight gain. In women, visceral fat can impact sex hormone levels. Overweight or obese women often experience an increase in androgens (male sex hormones) and a decrease in sex hormone-binding globulin (SHBG). These hormonal imbalances can contribute to conditions such as polycystic ovary syndrome (PCOS) and irregular menstrual cycles.

Influence on the Hypothalamus-Pituitary-Adrenal (HPA) Axis: Visceral fat may affect the function of the HPA axis, which regulates the body's response to stress and the production of hormones like cortisol. Elevated cortisol levels, as observed in individuals with chronic stress and excess visceral fat, can further disrupt metabolic and hormonal equilibrium.

In summary, excess visceral fat can disrupt hormone regulation through its role as an active endocrine organ, releasing various molecules that impact hormone balance, appetite control, and metabolism. These hormonal imbalances can contribute to conditions such as insulin resistance, metabolic syndrome, PCOS, and other health concerns.

Visceral fat presents various additional health risks, including:

❖ Fatty Liver Disease: Visceral fat located near the portal vein can transfer harmful substances to the liver, leading to liver inflammation and non-alcoholic fatty liver disease (NAFLD). This fat is also strongly linked to heart disease due to the substances it releases, increasing the risk of atherosclerosis, heart attacks, and strokes.

❖ Respiratory Impact: Excessive visceral fat can hinder lung expansion, causing breathing difficulties, especially in overweight or obese individuals.

❖ Gastrointestinal Issues: Visceral fat can increase pressure on the stomach and intestines, leading to problems such as acid reflux and irritable bowel syndrome (IBS). Additionally, carrying excess visceral fat can result in poor posture, reduced mobility, and an increased risk of musculoskeletal issues.

It's important to note that the presence of visceral fat is not always correlated with one's appearance or body mass index (BMI). Even individuals who appear slender can have excess visceral fat. This underscores the importance of adopting a healthy lifestyle, including regular exercise and a balanced diet, to reduce the risks associated with visceral fat accumulation. In subsequent chapters, we will discuss factors contributing to the buildup of belly fat and practical ways to reduce its accumulation.

CHAPTER ONE

<u>Major causes of belly fat</u>

Having learned about what belly fat entails, let's now examine some factors and habits that put us at risk of developing this condition. In general, individuals who consistently consume more calories than they burn each day are more prone to gaining excess weight, including belly fat. Additionally, aging plays a role in this process, as people tend to lose muscle mass as they get older, which is particularly problematic for those leading a sedentary lifestyle.

Now, let's provide a general overview of some habits that lead to the accumulation of belly fat:

Poor Diet:
A comprehensive understanding of how a poor diet is connected to the accumulation of belly fat involves several key factors:

Excess Caloric Intake: This term refers to consuming more calories than your body requires for daily energy expenditure and basic metabolic functions. The human body has a specific calorie requirement to maintain its current weight and support vital functions like breathing, digestion, and circulation. When individuals consistently consume more calories than their bodies expend, these surplus calories are stored as fat, with a tendency to accumulate in the abdominal region.

Carbohydrates: Carbohydrates can be generally classified into different categories:

Simple Carbohydrates: These are sugars made up of one or two sugar units. Examples include glucose, fructose (found in fruits), and sucrose (table sugar, composed of glucose and fructose).

Natural vs. Added Sugars: Natural sugars occur naturally in foods, such as the sugars in fruit and milk. Added sugars, on the other hand, are sugars incorporated during food processing, often in the form of high-fructose corn syrup, sucrose, or other sweeteners.

Complex Carbohydrates: Refined carbohydrates are complex carbohydrates that have undergone extensive processing, which removes most of their natural fiber and nutrients. Common sources include white bread, white rice, and pasta. These refined carbohydrates contribute to belly fat through several mechanisms:

❖ Refined carbohydrates have a high glycemic index, leading to rapid spikes in blood sugar levels, resulting in energy crashes and increased hunger and cravings shortly after consumption. The refining process removes the fiber found in whole grains, which aids in digestion and blood sugar regulation. Without this fiber, they are less satiating, promoting swift digestion and absorption of sugars and refined carbs, leading to feelings of hunger and overeating, making it easier to consume excess calories that may be stored as fat, particularly in the abdominal region.

❖ Excessive and frequent consumption of sugars and refined carbs can lead to insulin resistance, a condition where cells don't respond effectively to insulin, making it more challenging for the body to regulate blood sugar levels. In response, the body produces more insulin, potentially promoting fat storage, especially around the abdomen. Overproduction of insulin can lead to a spike in the conversion of excess glucose into fat, a process known as lipogenesis. This stored fat often concentrates in the abdominal area, contributing to abdominal obesity.

❖ Excessive sugar consumption, notably fructose found in high-fructose corn syrup, can contribute to the accumulation of fat in the liver (non-alcoholic fatty liver disease), which is associated with abdominal obesity.

In summary, a poor diet characterized by excess caloric intake, especially from refined carbohydrates and sugars, can significantly contribute to the accumulation of belly fat.

Processed and Trans Fats: Understanding how processed and trans fats influence the buildup of belly fat is crucial for maintaining good health. Processed fats undergo chemical and industrial processes to enhance their shelf life, taste, or texture. They often include hydrogenated and partially hydrogenated oils, interesterified fats, and other altered forms of natural fats. Trans fats, with a unique molecular structure due to hydrogenation, can occur naturally in small amounts in some animal products, but most health concerns surround artificial trans fats. They've been associated with unfavorable changes in lipid profiles, leading to abdominal fat storage and insulin resistance. Trans fats also elevate "bad" Low-Density Lipoprotein cholesterol levels and lower "good" High-Density Lipoprotein cholesterol levels, promoting abdominal fat accumulation and related health issues.

The combination of processed and trans fats can disrupt metabolic processes, causing hormonal imbalances that encourage abdominal fat storage. They can also trigger chronic inflammation, linked to visceral fat accumulation and related health problems.

Poor Fiber Intake: Another unhealthy dietary habit is consuming food poor in dietary fiber. Dietary fiber, found in plant-based foods like fruits, vegetables, whole grains, legumes, and nuts, is a type of carbohydrate not digested by the body. It creates a sense of fullness and satisfaction, helping control appetite and reducing the inclination to consume excessive calories and snacks, especially at night. Diets lacking in fiber tend to be less satisfying, leading to overeating and higher calorie consumption. Fiber aids in regulating blood sugar levels by slowing sugar absorption from the digestive tract. Hence, insufficient fiber intake can lead to rapid blood sugar spikes followed by crashes, triggering cravings and overeating, contributing to abdominal fat gain. Additionally, a deficiency in fiber can lead to constipation and digestive discomfort, potentially causing bloating and a distended belly, which might be mistaken for fat accumulation.

Low Protein Consumption: Yet another unhealthy diet habit is consuming food that's low in protein. Proteins, composed of amino acids, play a crucial role in bodily functions, tissue repair, and growth. They have a higher thermic effect, meaning your body expends more energy digesting them compared to fats or carbs. Adequate protein supports an efficient metabolism, helping burn calories instead of storing them as fat, which is vital for weight control. When protein is lacking, people may rely more on carbohydrates and fats. Protein-rich foods help curb hunger and reduce cravings, so a lack of protein in our diet may lead to increased appetite, often resulting in overeating and the consumption of calorie-dense, unhealthy foods, contributing to belly fat. Additionally, a protein deficiency can cause muscle loss, slowing metabolism and increasing weight gain.

Excessive Alcohol Consumption: This is another risk factor for belly fat. Alcohol is consumed for various reasons, such as socializing, relaxation, celebrations, and cultural traditions. Common alcoholic beverages include beer, wine, and spirits like vodka or whiskey. It's important to recognize that moderate alcohol consumption is generally considered acceptable and can even have potential health benefits. Moderate consumption is typically defined as one drink per day for women and up to two drinks per day for men. The definition of a "drink" varies based on the type of alcohol but is generally equivalent to 12 ounces of beer, 5 ounces of wine, or 1.5 ounces of distilled spirits. However, excessive or irresponsible drinking can have adverse effects on both physical and mental health.

This is due to the fact that alcohol is relatively calorie-dense, with each gram providing seven calories, making it second only to fat in terms of calorie density. Hence, consuming alcohol increases your calorie intake, potentially leading to weight gain. Alcohol can also stimulate appetite and lower inhibitions, which can result in overeating and an easier consumption of excess calories, often in the form of unhealthy snacks and meals. Moreover, when you consume alcohol, your body prioritizes metabolizing it over other macronutrients. This means that, temporarily, your body stops burning fat for energy, potentially resulting in fat storage, most especially in the abdominal area. Alcohol can also disrupt hormones that control appetite and fat storage, potentially increasing the likelihood of accumulating fat in the abdominal region.

As you must have heard before, excessive alcohol consumption can lead to liver damage, including a condition called non-alcoholic fatty liver disease (NAFLD), which can contribute to the accumulation of abdominal fat. Also, chronic alcohol consumption can lead to insulin resistance, which may promote abdominal obesity and raise the risk of type 2 diabetes. It can also elevate cortisol levels, a stress hormone associated with storing fat in the abdominal area.

Sedentary Lifestyle: This is another risk factor that plays a vital role in belly fat accumulation. A sedentary lifestyle involves prolonged sitting or lying down with little to no physical activity, a common occurrence in our modern, technology-driven world, where people spend extended hours at desks, in front of screens, or in vehicles. Inactivity leads to a decrease in daily calorie expenditure. When you don't use energy through movement, surplus calories are more likely to be stored as fat, especially around the abdomen. This type of lifestyle can lead to muscle atrophy, where muscles shrink and weaken due to a lack of use. Muscle tissue is more metabolically active than fat, so its loss can slow metabolism, making it easier to gain weight and accumulate abdominal fat.

Excessive Stress: On the opposite end of a sedentary lifestyle, we have excessive stress, and both can be at extreme points. Stress is the body's natural response to perceived threats or challenges and can result from various factors, including work pressure, financial concerns, personal relationships, and health issues. During excessive stress, cortisol, often known as the "stress hormone," is produced by the adrenal glands and plays various roles in the body. While it's essential for many functions, excessive cortisol production due to chronic stress can lead to the buildup of abdominal fat. Cortisol promotes fat storage, particularly visceral fat around abdominal organs. It can also relocate fat from other body areas to the abdomen. In addition, elevated cortisol levels can contribute to insulin resistance, increasing insulin levels and further promoting fat storage in the abdominal region. Excessive stress often leads to emotional eating or heightened cravings for calorie-rich foods as a way to find comfort, and consuming these high-calorie, sugary, or fatty foods as a coping mechanism can result in weight gain, particularly around the midsection. Chronic stress can also disrupt sleep patterns, and insufficient sleep has been generally associated with weight gain.

Hormonal Imbalances: This is another factor to consider regarding belly fat. Some individuals are often perplexed as to what brings about their weight gain even when they eat moderately and engage in several strenuous exercises. Hormonal imbalances, which are common, especially in women, can play a role in the buildup of belly fat. Hormones are vital chemical messengers regulating various bodily functions, including metabolism and fat storage, within the complex endocrine system.

Some factors contributing to hormonal imbalances

- ❖ Age: Hormone levels naturally fluctuate with age. In women, menopause is linked to a significant decline in estrogen and progesterone, potentially leading to abdominal fat gain.
- ❖ Stress: Chronic stress can disrupt hormonal balance by increasing the production of stress hormones like cortisol, which can promote abdominal obesity.
- ❖ Medical Conditions: Certain medical conditions, such as polycystic ovary syndrome (PCOS), thyroid disorders (hypothyroidism), Cushing's Syndrome, and insulin resistance, can disrupt hormonal balance.

❖ Medications: Some medications can affect hormone levels and how fat is distributed in the body. For instance, medications like antipsychotics, antidepressants, and corticosteroids may lead to weight gain as a side effect.

Examples of some common hormones and their negative impacts on the accumulation of belly fat include:

❖ Insulin: This hormone is produced by the pancreas, and it regulates blood sugar levels and how the body metabolizes carbohydrates, fats, and protein. When insulin is dysregulated due to issues like insulin resistance or excessive carbohydrate intake, it promotes the storage of glucose as fat, particularly in the form of visceral fat around abdominal organs. Additionally, as mentioned earlier, insulin resistance leads to a redistribution of fat, favoring storage in the abdominal area.

❖ Estrogen: This hormone has a protective role in determining how fat is distributed in the body. During menopause, which is a natural transition for women typically occurring between ages 45 and 55, there's usually a decrease in estrogen levels, and this decline is associated with an increased tendency to store fat in the abdominal region.

❖ Leptin: Also known as the "satiety hormone," it is produced by fat cells and communicates with the brain, providing information about the body's energy reserves. In a healthy state, rising leptin levels signal the brain to reduce appetite and increase energy expenditure. However, leptin resistance can develop, especially in cases of obesity, where the brain no longer effectively responds to leptin, leading to increased appetite and overeating, including cravings for high-calorie and sugary foods. Additionally, when leptin signaling is disrupted, the body may be more inclined to store fat, particularly in visceral fat deposits, such as abdominal fat.

Genetics: This is another factor that plays a vital role in fat distribution in the body. Genetics significantly contribute to determining an individual's body shape and how fat is distributed, including the likelihood of accumulating abdominal fat. While genes don't singlehandedly determine one's susceptibility to abdominal obesity, they do influence various factors that contribute to it. Our genes, which constitute our DNA, contain instructions for shaping and maintaining our bodies, and genetic differences among individuals can affect how the body stores and utilizes fat. Genes can impact an individual's basal metabolic rate (BMR) and how efficiently the body burns calories. Some people may possess genes that result in a higher BMR, making it easier for them to maintain a healthy weight, while others may have a slower BMR, which can lead to weight gain. Genes can also determine where the body tends to store fat. Some individuals may have a genetic predisposition to store fat in the abdominal area, leading to the accumulation of belly fat. Additionally, genetic factors can affect appetite, food preferences, and the regulation of hunger and fullness, which, in turn, can impact calorie intake and how fat is stored. In the next chapter, we will be looking at the main purpose of this book which is ' the practical ways of reducing belly fat'.

CHAPTER TWO

Evidence-based, practical strategies for reducing abdominal fat

Luckily, there are several strategies for reducing belly fat, which lowers your risk of developing a variety of diseases connected to excessive body fat. Here are some research-backed strategies for reducing belly fat:

Healthy diet: This involves adopting a balanced, nutrient-rich eating pattern that promotes overall well-being and lowers the risk of chronic diseases. It provides the body with the essential elements it needs to perform at its best. This approach focuses on portion control and balanced nutrition to reduce abdominal fat. Below is a comprehensive overview of the main concepts behind these diets and practical ways to maintain them:

Calorie Deficit Diets: These diets are regimens of food designed to consistently lower energy intake in order to encourage weight loss. The ideas of calories and calorie deficit diets are foundational to both weight management and nutrition. Generally, energy is measured in calories. That is, a calorie is a unit of measurement used in nutrition that indicates how much energy your body gets from a specific food or beverage. Your daily caloric intake is the total quantity of calories you consume from all the foods and drinks you have during the day. The quantity of calories in various foods varies. For instance, compared to proteins and carbs, which have roughly 4 calories per gram each, fats have approximately 9 calories per gram. A calorie deficit is the state in which your body uses more calories than it takes in. It's a cornerstone of losing weight. Basically, during this state, the body begins to use stored energy, usually in the form of body fat, to make up for the energy deficit. This causes you to lose weight, which, in turn, lessens abdominal fat. These practices typically involve monitoring your calorie intake, either by counting calories or controlling portions, to ensure you consume fewer calories than your body requires for daily activities and metabolism. It doesn't limit specific foods but focuses on reducing overall calorie intake.

How to follow and sustain calorie deficit diet:

❖ Calculate your daily caloric needs, known as Total Daily Energy Expenditure (TDEE), which includes your Basal Metabolic Rate (BMR) and calories burned through physical activity. This will guide you in determining the amount of calories you need per day.

❖ Make gradual changes to your diet. Avoid sudden, drastic alterations as they can be hard to maintain. Small, sustainable adjustments are more likely to become long-term habits.

❖ Set a realistic goal for yourself: By aiming for a moderate calorie loss per day, usually between 500 to 1,000 calories below your TDEE per day, which can result in gradual and consistent weight loss of about 1 to 2 pounds every week.

❖ Keep track of your calorie intake: Using apps, food diaries, or labels to ensure you stay within your calorie deficit. Always try to avoid emotional or stress-related overeating by paying rapt attention to your body's signals of hunger and fullness.

❖ Plan your meals and snacks in advance to avoid impulsive, high-calorie choices. Ensure a well-balanced mix of nutrients. Regularly monitor changes in weight, body measurements, or body composition to stay motivated and make necessary adjustments.

❖ Nutrient-based food: Opt for foods rich in nutrients. Choose nutrient-packed foods that supply vital vitamins and minerals. This not only promotes general well-being but also makes you feel more satisfied with fewer calories. Give priority to whole, unprocessed foods such as lean proteins, whole grains, fruits, vegetables, and healthy fats. These foods offer essential nutrients while managing calorie intake.

When it comes to calorie deficit diets, it's crucial to maintain a sense of equilibrium and caution. Excessive calorie restriction can be detrimental and unsustainable. Remember that maintaining a calorie deficit diet is an ongoing process rather than a final goal. It's about developing long-lasting, healthful behaviors that you can stick with. Practice self-compassion and concentrate on making little, steady improvements rather than rushing to solutions. Most importantly, remain adaptable and willing to modify your plan if you encounter plateaus or challenges. Adaptation is a part of achieving long-term success.

Balanced Macronutrients: This is another means of reducing your belly fat as regards your diet. A well-rounded intake of macronutrients is vital for overall health and can play a significant role in reducing abdominal fat when combined with a holistic approach to weight management. Macronutrients are the primary nutrients that supply the body with substantial energy, and a balanced consumption of these macronutrients supports various bodily functions and contributes to reducing belly fat. These macronutrients include:

Carbohydrates: These are a fundamental macronutrient that provides the body with energy. When consumed appropriately within a balanced diet and lifestyle, carbohydrates can support overall health and assist in reducing belly fat.

Types of Carbohydrates:
* Complex carbs: Foods such as fruits, vegetables, legumes, and whole grains contain complex carbs. In addition to being high in fiber, vitamins, and minerals, these carbohydrates offer a consistent energy delivery that lowers blood sugar levels.
* Simple Carbohydrates:** Simple carbohydrates are found in foods like sugary snacks, candies, and sugary beverages. They are often high in added sugars and provide a quick but short-lived source of energy.

What is the best approach to carbohydrate consumption for reduction of belly fat?

Prioritize Whole Foods: Choose complex carbohydrates from whole foods like brown rice, quinoa, oats, and vegetables. These foods are rich in fiber and nutrients, and they provide a steady slow release of glucose, preventing rapid spikes and crashes in blood sugar levels. This is important for reducing cravings and overeating, which can lead to abdominal fat gain.

Limit Sugary and Refined Carbohydrates: Minimize or avoid sugary snacks, sweets, and sugary beverages. These can lead to increased belly fat when consumed in excess due to rapid blood sugar fluctuations. Consume carbohydrates as part of a balanced diet that includes a variety of macronutrients. That is, balance your carbohydrate intake with proteins and healthy fats.

Prioritize Fiber: Choose high-fiber carbohydrates like whole grains, legumes, and vegetables to support satiety and digestive health. Furthermore, distribute your carbohydrate intake evenly throughout the day to maintain steady blood sugar levels and prevent overeating during later meals. Lastly, be mindful of portion sizes when consuming carbohydrates to avoid excessive calorie intake.

Proteins: Proteins are a fundamental macronutrient essential for various physiological functions in the body. They play a vital role in reducing belly fat through the following mechanisms:

❖ Satiety: Proteins have a stronger satiating effect, helping you feel full and satisfied. This can reduce overall calorie intake and minimize overeating, which is crucial for weight loss, including the loss of abdominal fat.

❖ Muscle Preservation: Adequate protein intake is essential for preserving and building lean muscle mass. More muscle means a higher resting metabolic rate, which can help burn more calories and reduce belly fat over time.

❖ Thermic Effect: Proteins have a higher thermic effect compared to carbohydrates and fats. They need more energy for metabolism and digestion, which increases calorie expenditure. Additionally, eating protein together with carbohydrates helps balance blood sugar levels, reducing energy spikes and crashes that can trigger overindulgence and cravings.

When including proteins in your diet, opt for lean sources like poultry, fish, lean meat, tofu, tempeh, legumes, and low-fat dairy products. Prioritize whole foods over processed protein sources because whole foods provide a variety of essential nutrients that can aid your overall health and weight loss efforts. Reduce your intake of red and processed meats, as excessive consumption of these is linked to health risks. It's vital to combine proteins with a generous portion of non-starchy vegetables to boost fiber intake, promote a feeling of fullness, and support your digestive health. Additionally, ensure you stay well-hydrated by drinking enough water when consuming protein, as it aids in digestion and prevents dehydration, which can sometimes be mistaken for hunger.

Fats: Fats, also known as lipids, are a group of organic molecules that serve diverse essential functions in the body. They are a complex macronutrient with various roles and can influence the accumulation of belly fat. It's crucial to consume fats wisely for effective belly fat reduction and overall weight management.

There are two main categories of fats:

Healthy Fats:
Monounsaturated Fats (MUFAs): Monounsaturated fats are a type of dietary fat that promotes heart health when consumed in moderation and can contribute to reducing belly fat as part of a balanced diet. They are identified by their chemical structure, featuring a single unsaturated carbon-carbon bond in their fatty acid chains. MUFAs are usually liquid at room temperature and solidify when refrigerated. You can find them in foods like avocados, olive oil, nuts, and seeds.

Polyunsaturated Fats (PUFAs): Polyunsaturated fats, similar to MUFAs, are beneficial for health when consumed in moderation. They are distinguished by having multiple unsaturated carbon-carbon bonds in their fatty acid chains. These fats are typically liquid at room temperature and are present in various foods and oils. They include two primary categories: omega-3 and omega-6 fatty acids, each offering unique health advantages. You can find them in fatty fish (such as salmon and mackerel), flaxseeds, walnuts, and certain vegetable oils. Omega-3 fatty acids, in particular, can reduce inflammation and enhance insulin sensitivity, contributing to the reduction of belly fat.

Unhealthy Fats:
Saturated Fats: Saturated fats are a type of dietary fat commonly found in various foods, predominantly from animal sources and some plant-based items. They are recognized by their chemical structure, where carbon atoms are completely "saturated" with hydrogen atoms, resulting in a stable and straight molecular arrangement. Saturated fats are typically solid at room temperature and are considered less healthy when consumed excessively. You can typically find them in fatty cuts of meat, full-fat dairy products, and certain plant oils like coconut oil. Consuming high amounts of saturated fats, especially from animal origins, is linked to an increase in belly fat and should be limited.

Trans Fats: Trans fats, also known as trans fatty acids, are a type of dietary fat artificially created through a chemical process called hydrogenation. This process involves adding hydrogen to liquid vegetable oils to make them solid at room temperature. Trans fats have a distinct chemical structure, where hydrogen atoms are on opposite sides of carbon-carbon double bonds, resulting in a "trans" configuration. They have been widely used in the food industry to improve the texture, shelf life, and taste of processed foods. However, they have been associated with significant negative health impacts, including increased abdominal fat. Furthermore, trans fats are strongly linked to a higher risk of heart disease. They raise levels of "bad" LDL cholesterol while reducing "good" HDL cholesterol in the bloodstream, both of which are risk factors for heart disease.

Due to their adverse health effects, many countries have instituted regulations to restrict or ban the use of trans fats in the food industry. For example, in the United States, the Food and Drug Administration (FDA) determined that partially hydrogenated oils (the primary source of artificial trans fats) are not "generally recognized as safe" and prohibited their use in foods. Health organizations like the World Health Organization (WHO) and the American Heart Association recommend minimizing trans fat intake as much as possible. Hence, it's essential to scrutinize food labels for trans fat content and make informed choices to avoid products containing partially hydrogenated oils. A diet low in trans fats promotes better heart health and overall well-being.

In summary, when incorporating fat into a well-balanced diet, choose sources of healthy fats, such as avocados, olive oil, nuts, seeds, and fatty fish like salmon. These fats are associated with reduced abdominal fat. Simultaneously, limit the consumption of saturated and trans fats as much as possible.

Fruits and Vegetables: Fruits and vegetables are crucial components of a healthy diet and play a significant role in managing weight, including reducing belly fat. They offer several advantages in terms of body weight:

Contributions of fruits and vegetables to belly fat reduction:

❖ Low in Calories: Fruits and vegetables are generally low in calories but rich in nutrients, making them excellent choices for weight loss.

❖ Abundant in Fiber: They serve as a great source of dietary fiber, which promotes a feeling of fullness, reducing overall calorie consumption. Additionally, many fruits and vegetables, like watermelon and cucumber, have high water content, aiding in hydration and satiety.

❖ Nutrient-Rich: Fruits and vegetables provide essential vitamins, minerals, and antioxidants that support overall health and metabolism. They also contain natural sugars, offering a sweet taste without causing spikes in blood sugar levels.

While they offer these essential nutrients, overconsumption can still lead to excessive calorie intake. Therefore, be mindful of portion sizes and diversify your fruit and vegetable choices to ensure a broad spectrum of nutrients and antioxidants.

Limiting Alcohol: Excessive alcohol consumption, as discussed in the previous chapter, can lead to the accumulation of belly fat. Hence, if you are committed to losing belly fat, consider reducing or eliminating alcohol from your diet for a period. The relationship between alcohol and weight loss is complex and varies from person to person. While moderate alcohol intake can fit into a balanced diet, excessive or frequent consumption is generally counterproductive to weight loss goals, especially for losing belly fat. If you must take alcohol, drink with moderation. The key is to restrict your intake to avoid excess calories. Opt for lower-calorie, lower-sugar alcoholic beverages like light beer, wine (in moderation), and spirits with low-calorie mixers. Avoid pairing alcohol with high-calorie snacks or fast food, as this can hinder your weight loss efforts. Lastly, avoid drinking on an empty stomach. Eating a balanced meal before drinking can slow alcohol absorption and mitigate its impact on blood sugar levels. In the upcoming chapter, we will delve into exercise as another essential tool for losing belly fat.

CHAPTER THREE

<u>Exercise and its contributions to belly fat reduction</u>

"Exercise is your king, and nutrition is your queen. Together, they create your fitness kingdom." - Jack LaLanne

Exercise involves planned, structured, and repetitive physical activities aimed at enhancing or sustaining physical fitness, general well-being, or specific fitness objectives. It is a foundational element of a healthy lifestyle and plays a vital role in reducing belly fat. Exercise can be categorized into various types based on their focus, intensity, and purpose. These include;

Cardiovascular or Aerobic Exercises: Cardiovascular exercise, often known as "cardio," encompasses physical activities specifically designed to target and enhance the cardiovascular system, including the heart and blood vessels. These exercises are typically aerobic, involving continuous, rhythmic movements that elevate your heart rate and breathing. They challenge your cardiovascular system, requiring your heart and lungs to work harder. The primary aim of cardiovascular exercise is to enhance cardiovascular health, boost endurance, and foster overall fitness. Importantly, cardio exercises burn calories, making them effective for weight management and reducing belly fat. The number of calories burned depends on exercise intensity. Examples of cardio activities include running, dancing, jogging, cycling, swimming, and brisk walking.

Strength or Resistance Training: Resistance exercise is a form of physical activity concentrated on working against resistance to enhance muscle strength, endurance, and overall physical fitness. The primary objective of resistance training is to increase the force or load on your muscles, compelling them to contract and adapt to become stronger. While resistance exercises don't directly target belly fat, they play a crucial role in building muscle and elevating metabolism, contributing to overall fat loss, particularly in the abdominal region, especially for men.

Notable examples of resistance exercises that aid in reducing belly fat;

Squats: Squats are a popular form of resistance exercise known for targeting the muscles of the lower body, including the quadriceps, hamstrings, glutes, and calves. While it's important to note that squats don't directly lead to the reduction of belly fat, they do play a crucial role in a comprehensive weight loss and fat-reduction program.

Executing squats correctly is paramount to prevent injury and maximize their benefits. Here's a step-by-step guide on how to perform a basic bodyweight squat, which serves as an excellent starting point:

❖ Stand Tall: Commence by standing with your feet positioned shoulder-width apart. Ensure your chest is up, shoulders are back, and you're looking straight ahead.
❖ Initiate the Movement: Begin the squat by pushing your hips back, simulating the action of sitting in a chair. This initial movement should primarily involve your hips and not your knees.
❖ Bend Your Knees: As you push your hips backward, gradually begin to bend your knees while maintaining proper alignment with your feet. It's crucial to avoid allowing your knees to extend beyond your toes.
❖ Lower Yourself: Continue lowering your body by bending both your hips and knees until your thighs are parallel to the ground. Your body weight should

be distributed over your heels, and your back should remain in a straight, upright position.

* ❖ Maintain Proper Form: Pay attention to keeping your chest up, your back straight, and engage your core muscles. This not only ensures good form but also contributes to stability during the exercise.
* ❖ Stand Up: Push through your heels and straighten your hips and knees to return to the starting position.
* ❖ Repeat: Carry out the squat for your desired number of times. For beginners, a reasonable starting point might be 2-3 sets of 10-15 reps, with gradual increases as you become more comfortable with the movement.

Tips for Proper Squat Form:

1. Throughout the entire exercise, keep your feet firm on the ground.
2. Prevent your knees from collapsing inward and ensure they remain in line with your feet.
3. Maintain an upright chest and avoid any rounding or arching of your lower back.
4. Always engage your core muscles to enhance stability.
5. Be mindful of your breathing: Inhale as you lower yourself into the squat and exhale as you push back up.

Once you have become proficient with bodyweight squats, you can introduce resistance by using dumbbells, a barbell, or a squat rack. Additionally, there are various squat variations, such as goblet squats, front squats, or single-leg squats, which can add variety and challenge to your workout routine.

It is imperative to prioritize proper form and technique over the amount of weight or the number of repetitions. If you are new to squats or strength training, it is advisable to consider working with a fitness professional to ensure that you are performing the exercise safely and effectively.

Another highly effective resistance exercise for reducing belly fat is the "Kettlebell Swing." Here are the steps to perform this exercise:

❖ Starting Position: Begin by standing with your feet shoulder-width apart, with your toes slightly pointed outward. Place a kettlebell down on the floor in front of you.

❖ Grip the Kettlebell: Bend at your hips and knees while maintaining a straight back. Reach for the kettlebell with both hands, gripping the handle with an overhand grip. Extend your arms, engaging your core, and set your shoulder blades back and down. Your back should stay straight, and your hips should be higher than your knees.

❖ Swinging Movement: Swing the kettlebell back between your legs while taking a breath. Keeping your arms straight, exhale hard as you drive the kettlebell forward to your shoulder height by thrusting your hips forward. To finish the workout, swing the kettlebell back and forth between your legs.

❖ Repetition: Continue performing the kettlebell swing for your desired number of repetitions. This dynamic exercise involves a hip-hinging motion and engages the core, glutes, hamstrings, and lower back.

Tips for Kettlebell Swings:
1) Utilize your hips to generate the movement's power, rather than relying on your arms. The swing is primarily a hip-dominant exercise.
2) Maintain a neutral spine with a straight back throughout the entire movement.
3) Keep your core activated to ensure stability and protect your lower back.

4) Begin with an appropriate weight for your fitness level and progressively increase it as you become more accustomed to the exercise.

5) The kettlebell swing is a high-intensity exercise; correct form is crucial to prevent injury.

Kettlebell swings are effective for calorie burning, core strengthening, and engaging multiple muscle groups, making them an excellent choice for overall fat loss, including the reduction of belly fat. As with any exercise, consistency and a well-balanced diet are essential for achieving significant results. Just like I said earlier, if you're new to kettlebell swings or resistance training, it's advisable to seek guidance from a fitness professional or personal trainer to ensure proper form and safety.

Other resistance exercises that can contribute to your fitness routine include planks, lunges, push-ups, Bent-over Rows, and more. To effectively incorporate these exercises, focus on full-body workouts targeting various muscle groups. Gradually increasing resistance or weight is crucial to continually challenge your muscles. Additionally, combine strength training with cardiovascular exercise and maintain a balanced diet for a holistic approach to losing belly fat and achieving your fitness goals.

High-Intensity Interval Training (HIIT): This is a widely popular and effective cardiovascular exercise method characterized by brief, vigorous bursts of activity followed by short periods of rest or low-intensity exercise. HIIT stands out as a significant contributor to the reduction of belly fat and overall fat loss. Here's a detailed explanation of how HIIT operates and its role in fat reduction, especially concerning belly fat:

- ❖ High Intensity: The high-intensity phase of HIIT involves giving near-maximum effort in activities such as sprinting or jumping, rapidly elevating your heart rate. Typically, high-intensity intervals in HIIT are short, typically ranging from 20 seconds to 2 minutes.
- ❖ Recovery Period: Following the high-intensity phase, a brief recovery period is introduced, where you either rest or engage in low-intensity activities like walking or slow cycling.
- ❖ Repetition: Multiple cycles of high-intensity and recovery intervals are repeated within a single HIIT session, making it a time-efficient exercise choice.

Roles of HIIT in Reducing Belly Fat:

Calorie Expenditure: HIIT is exceptionally efficient at burning calories, even within a short time frame.

The intense efforts significantly boost heart rate and metabolism, leading to a substantial calorie burn. It also triggers what is known as Excess Post-Exercise Oxygen Consumption (EPOC), often referred to as the "afterburn effect." This means your body continues to burn calories at an elevated rate even after you've finished exercising, contributing to overall fat loss. EPOC can extend for hours or even days. Hence, it has demonstrated the ability to enhance the body's capacity to burn fat for energy, a crucial factor in shedding stored fat, including belly fat. It is known for its tendency to preserve muscle mass while promoting fat loss, a vital aspect for maintaining a healthy metabolism.

Improved Insulin Sensitivity: HIIT can enhance insulin sensitivity, regulating blood sugar levels and reducing the risk of fat accumulation in the abdominal region. Additionally, HIIT sessions are often shorter compared to traditional steady-state cardio exercises, yet they deliver equivalent or superior results when it comes to fat loss.

Here's an uncomplicated example of a HIIT workout that you can engage in:

❖ Warm-up: Start with 5 minutes of light aerobic exercise, such as jogging in place or doing jumping jacks.

❖ High-Intensity Phase: For 30 seconds, either sprint or perform a demanding activity like high knees.

❖ Recovery Phase: Take it easy by walking or jogging at a slower pace for 30-60 seconds.

❖ Repeat: Go through the high-intensity and recovery phases 5-10 times.

❖ Cool Down: Conclude with 5 minutes of light aerobic exercise and incorporate some stretching.

In summary, HIIT's distinct approach to cardiovascular exercise through high-intensity intervals and strategic recovery periods makes it an exceptional choice for individuals aiming to reduce belly fat and achieve comprehensive fat loss. It is important to choose HIIT exercises that you find enjoyable, safe, and sustainable.

Core Strengthening Exercises: These exercises are crucial for the development and maintenance of a robust and steady core, encompassing the muscles in your abdomen, lower back, hips, and pelvis. While core exercises don't directly burn belly fat, they exert a notable impact on your overall fitness and weight loss journey. A good example is the plank exercise.

Method:

* Begin in a push-up position with your elbows positioned directly under your shoulders.**
* Keep your body in a straight line from your head to your heels, thereby utilizing your core.**
* Sustain this posture for as long as you can uphold proper form.**

By incorporating core-strengthening exercises like the plank into your fitness routine, you'll build a solid foundation for overall fitness, complementing your HIIT workouts and contributing to your weight loss goals.

Roles of Exercises in Reducing Belly Fat:

Calorie Expenditure: Both cardiovascular exercises and HIIT routines help in calorie burning, creating a calorie deficit that can result in overall fat reduction, including belly fat. Furthermore, strength training and HIIT can raise muscle mass, elevating your resting metabolic rate and promoting calorie burn, even at rest.

Targeted Core Enhancement: Core exercises serve to fortify and sculpt the abdominal muscles, potentially contributing to a more toned and defined waistline. Additionally, physical activity has the ability to reduce stress, known for its association with the accumulation of abdominal fat. And as we all know, reduced stress levels can be beneficial for belly fat reduction.

Hormonal Regulation: Exercise plays a part in the regulation of hormones associated with fat storage and appetite, potentially reducing belly fat. Furthermore, regular exercise provides numerous health benefits, reducing the risk of chronic ailments like diabetes and heart disease, which are linked to abdominal obesity.

Effective Strategies for Reducing Belly Fat through Exercise

❖ Blend Cardio and Strength Training: The most effective approach to reducing belly fat involves a combination of both aerobic and strength exercises.
❖ Consistency: Consistently adhering to your exercise regimen is paramount. Strive for at least 150 minutes of moderate-intensity exercise or 75 minutes of vigorous-intensity exercise each week and complement your exercise routine with a healthy and well-balanced diet to optimize your results. Also, Staying well-hydrated is vital for supporting metabolic processes and overall well-being.

In conclusion, exercises encompass a wide array of approaches, each with a significant role in reducing belly fat by burning calories, building muscle, and fostering holistic health. A comprehensive strategy that integrates diverse exercise types with a balanced diet and healthful lifestyle choices is the most effective path to realize your desired outcomes. Seeking advice from a fitness expert or personal trainer can help in formulating a customized exercise plan aligned with your objectives. In the next chapter, we will discuss gut bacteria and how to take advantage of the knowledge of their roles in the body to reduce weight gain and, by extension, belly fat.

CHAPTER FOUR

Gut Bacteria and Belly Fat

For a century, we've known that bacteria reside in our intestines, but our understanding was that they played a minimal role in our health. We believed they merely thrived on the warmth and nutrients in our gut. In the last decade, significant breakthroughs have allowed scientists to quantify and characterize the genes found in our gut bacteria. The findings have been astonishing. Our gut bacteria possess 250 to 800 times more genes than we do as humans. Even more remarkable, these bacterial genes produce substances that enter our bloodstream, influencing our body chemistry. This suggests that the bacteria in our gut might indeed impact our health.

How then can they influence our weight? When we consume food, our gut breaks it down into small components. Only the tiniest particles are absorbed into our bloodstream, while the rest is expelled as waste. In other words, not all the calories from the food we eat enter our bodies and contribute to our weight. Gut bacteria play a role in breaking down food, and some bacteria are more adept at breaking it down into those tiny particles that can be digested, adding calories to our bodies and potentially leading to weight gain. In theory, if our guts harbor a greater quantity of these bacteria, it might be more challenging to lose weight.

But is there concrete evidence to support this theory? Of course! Several studies in animals, as well as some involving humans, suggest that this may indeed be the case. For instance, scientists conducted experiments where they transferred bacteria from the intestines of two strains of mice - one that naturally became obese and another that naturally remained lean - into a third strain of lean mice that were raised without any gut bacteria from birth. The gut bacteria transferred from naturally obese mice caused the germ-free mice to become overweight, whereas those transferred from the naturally lean mice kept them slender.

Subsequently, scientists conducted experiments where they extracted bacteria from the intestines of human identical twins, one of whom was obese and the other lean. They then transplanted these bacteria into the intestines of lean, germ-free mice. Notably, bacteria from the obese twin caused the mice to gain weight, while bacteria from the lean twin did not yield the same effect.

Our comprehension of the role of gut bacteria in obesity is in its early stages, and as of now, this scientific knowledge has not yet led to treatments that facilitate weight loss. Regardless, the correlation between gut bacteria and abdominal fat has emerged as a prominent subject within the realm of health and nutrition. This connection primarily revolves around the gut microbiome, which encompasses the multitude of microorganisms residing within our digestive tract, including bacteria, viruses, and fungi. These microorganisms play an integral role in processes like digestion, nutrient absorption, and overall well-being.

The majority of these microorganisms are friendly bacteria that generate essential nutrients, such as certain B vitamins and vitamin K. They are also instrumental in breaking down dietary fiber, an indigestible component, converting it into valuable short-chain fatty acids like butyrate. Two principal categories of beneficial bacteria found in the gut are bacteroidetes and firmicutes. The balance between these two bacterial families appears to be linked to body weight, making an understanding of their roles crucial due to the substantial implications they hold for human health and metabolism.

Bacteroidetes: This is a prominent phylum within the human gut microbiota. They represent a diverse array of microorganisms. These bacteria are characterized by their gram-negative nature, lack of spore-forming capability, and reliance on anaerobic metabolism, thriving in oxygen-deprived environments. Their essential functions include maintaining gut health, contributing to digestion, and influencing various facets of human physiology. They are responsible for the breakdown of complex carbohydrates and dietary fibers and participate in the fermentation of non-digestible dietary fibers, resulting in the production of beneficial short-chain fatty acids (SCFAs), which are vital for gut health and energy metabolism.

An abundance of Bacteroidetes is typically associated with a healthy and diverse gut microbiome, and achieving a balanced ratio of Bacteroidetes to Firmicutes is considered an ideal state for upholding gut health and metabolic equilibrium.

Firmicutes: These constitute another significant phylum of bacteria in the gut, and they differ from Bacteroidetes as they are gram-positive and thrive in anaerobic conditions. Their defining characteristic is the thick, peptidoglycan-rich cell walls, which stain purple in Gram staining, setting them apart from Gram-negative bacteria. Firmicutes are adept fermenters of carbohydrates and play a pivotal role in extracting energy from the diet. Research has indicated a potential connection between the relative abundance of Firmicutes in the gut and conditions like obesity. Some findings suggest that individuals with obesity or higher body fat percentages may exhibit a greater proportion of Firmicutes in their gut microbiome. One proposed mechanism is the efficiency of Firmicutes in extracting calories from otherwise indigestible complex carbohydrates, ultimately leading to increased calorie intake and potential weight gain, including the accumulation of belly fat.

Strategies for Promoting Bacteroidetes and Supporting Weight Management

As I mentioned earlier, equilibrium between Firmicutes and Bacteroidetes in the gut microbiome holds a special place in research, particularly regarding weight management and the reduction of abdominal fat. While this relationship is intricate and varies among individuals, below are some strategies that might help elevate Bacteroidetes levels, potentially contributing to weight loss and the reduction of belly fat:

❖ Dietary Fiber: Elevate your consumption of dietary fiber, encompassing fruits, vegetables, whole grains, and legumes. Bacteroidetes thrive on fiber, which acts as a prebiotic, providing nourishment for this beneficial bacteria.

❖ Probiotics and Prebiotics:** Probiotics, comprising beneficial bacteria or yeasts like Lactobacillus and Bifidobacterium, can be found in foods such as yogurt, kefir, and fermented foods. They may promote a diverse gut microbiome. Additionally, certain probiotics are believed to influence appetite and energy utilization by producing short-chain fatty acids, which might inhibit dietary fat absorption, potentially resulting in fewer calories absorbed from food. Prebiotics, which are non-digestible dietary fibers, serve as a food source for beneficial gut bacteria, particularly probiotics. They encourage the growth and activity of these beneficial microorganisms in the gastrointestinal tract. Foods like garlic, onions, and leeks contain prebiotics and support the growth of Bacteroidetes and other beneficial bacteria.

❖ Reducing Saturated Fats: Limit your saturated fat and trans fat intake, as high-fat diets may favor the growth of Firmicutes over Bacteroidetes. Additionally, a balanced approach to protein intake is advisable, as high-protein diets can affect the composition of the gut microbiome.

In summary, the relationship between gut bacteria and abdominal fat is intricate and dynamic. Bacteroidetes and Firmicutes are two significant bacterial phyla in the human gut, each playing distinct roles in digestion, metabolism, and overall health. Achieving a balance between these phyla is crucial for a healthy gut microbiome and may have implications for weight management and metabolic well-being. A diverse and balanced gut microbiome can contribute to overall health and support a healthier body composition. Conversely, an imbalanced microbiome can lead to inflammation, insulin resistance, and increased abdominal fat. Incorporating a fiber-rich diet and beneficial bacteria can be a constructive step towards maintaining a healthy gut and potentially reducing belly fat, though individual responses may vary.

CHAPTER FIVE

SUMMARY

Losing belly fat requires a combination of a healthy lifestyle, which includes diet and exercise. Start by focusing on whole foods like fruits, vegetables, and whole grains, while always incorporating lean proteins such as chicken, fish, tofu, and more to help maintain muscle mass. Simultaneously, limit your intake of processed foods, sugary drinks, and high-calorie snacks, and make a conscious effort to control portion sizes and eat in moderation.

To achieve your goal, it's crucial to maintain a calorie deficit by consistently consuming fewer calories than you burn. Utilize a calorie tracker to monitor your intake and aim for a sustainable deficit. Staying well-hydrated with plenty of water will not only support your overall health but also help control your appetite.

Incorporate a well-rounded exercise regimen, including both aerobic (cardio) and strength training exercises. Endeavor to carryout not less than 150 minutes of moderate-intensity aerobic activity every week. Additionally, consider the effectiveness of High-Intensity Interval Training (HIIT) workouts, which can expedite calorie burning and reduce belly fat within a shorter timeframe.

Strengthening your core with exercises like planks, leg raises, and crunches is essential for achieving a toned midsection. Prioritize getting 7-9 hours of quality sleep each night to facilitate weight loss, and remember to manage stress effectively through techniques such as meditation or yoga.

Keep in mind that spot reduction (losing fat from a specific area) is a challenging endeavor, so focusing on overall weight loss and adopting a healthy lifestyle is the most effective approach to reduce belly fat over time.

Patience and consistency are key in this journey as it takes time to see noticeable results. If you have specific health concerns or find it challenging to lose belly fat, it's advisable to consult with a healthcare professional or a registered dietitian for personalized guidance.

Finally, thanks for buying and taking your time to read through this book. Did this book provide any benefit or help you in any way? If so, I'd be interested and happy to hear about it. Honest reviews assist other readers in finding the right book for their needs. Hence, please endeavor to rate and drop your reviews on how this book impacted your life, for doing so not only encourage us authors but also help other readers who might be looking for similar solutions to their problems. As you do so, may God bless and support you in your journey to losing weight and living a healthy lifestyle. Remain blessed!!!